Hemorrhoids naturally treated with Homeopathy and Schuessler salts (homeopathic cell salts)

Robert Kopf

Copyright © 2021 Robert Kopf

ISBN 9798752484353

CONTENT

INTRODUCTION

Robert Kopf, Author of Naturopathy and Traditional healer

Translated from german edition by the author

Hemorrhoids, also called piles, are swollen and inflamed veins located inside the rectum (internal hemorrhoids), or they may develop around the anus (external hemorrhoids). You can have both types at the same time.

The most common complaints are bleeding, itching and inflammation in the anal region, pain, swelling, leakage of feces and feeling a lump near the anus.

Hemorrhoids may result from straining during bowel movements, an increased pressure on the veins in the pelvic and rectal area, a weak connective tissue, sitting for long periods of time on the toilet, chronic diarrhea or constipation, liver disease, obesity, pregnancy and low-fiber diet.

In the homeopathic and biochemical treatment (Schuessler salts) of hemorrhoids, detoxification therapies serve the activation of metabolism, strengthening the blood vessels and connective tissue. It cleans, de-acidifies the body, is mineralizing and leads to a balanced life energy.

The body will be purified and the dissolved metabolic waste, acids and toxins are excreted through the intestines, urinary tract, lungs and skin.

Hemorrhoids can also be caused and reinforced by a mineral deficiency and an acidification of the body. Mineral deficiency and acidification in turn weaken the hormonal system, the connective tissue of the blood vessels and immune system.

Also a defective metabolism favors hemorrhoids, acidification and chronic health problems and is often the result of a disturbance of mineral intake and mineral distribution.

Although we may receive enough minerals in our food, in the event of a metabolic disorder, not all of the minerals may reach the cells.

The use of homeopathic remedies and Schuessler salts is a good way to compensate this mineral deficiency in a natural way and to treat and prevent hemorrhoids.

Stress, acidification of the body, as well as environmental toxins hinder the mineral transport through the cell membranes. This is where the effect of Homeopathy and Schuessler salts works.

They activate the excretion of toxins and acids. The basal metabolic rate increases and the self-healing power of the body is activated.

First I like to explain you the therapies for the treatment and prevention of hemorrhoids offered in this guide:

Homeopathy was developed about 200 years ago by Samuel Hahnemann. The three basic principles of Homeopathy are the simile rule, homeopathic drug testing and detection of individual disease.

The most important principle is the principle of similarity (simile rule), which was formulated in 1796 by Hahnemann.

It states that a patient should be treated with the remedy, which can cause in its original state similar symptoms in healthy people like the existing disease. It notes primarily the main complaints of the patient.

Together with a few differentiating additional informations (modalities) then the right remedy will be found for the treatment of hemorrhoids.

The dosage depends on the condition of the patient. As the patient improves, the distances between the medication will be gradually extended.

What happens if you choose the wrong remedy? Nothing - just as a key does not turn in the wrong door lock, a wrong homeopathic remedy does not cause any reaction in the body.

The homeopathic remedies are available as D-, C- and LM potencies.

For the beginners in Homeopathy, I recommend the use of lower D-potencies. Higher potencies (D200, C and LM potencies) should only be given by an expert, as they go very deep in their effects and are often used only once.

Schuessler salts (also named homeopathic cell salts, tissue salts, Biochemistry) for the treatment and prevention of hemorrhoids

In the 19th century the german physician Dr. Wilhelm Heinrich Schuessler (1821 to 1898) developed his health cure with homeopathic mineral salts. In recent years this therapy celebrated a comeback.

In his studies Schuessler discovered twelve mineral compounds, comprised each of a base and an acid, which play a crucial role in the function and structure of the body. He developed his own system with which many diseases can be treated in a natural way (also hemorrhoids).

Schuessler focused his search on mineral salts and trace elements, which are found in every cell of the body and called his method of healing "Biochemistry" (chemistry of life).

It is based on the assumption that nearly every disease is caused because of the lack of a specific mineral salt. This leads to dysregulations inside the cells. The molecules cannot flow freely.

A mineral salt deficiency arises from the fact that the cells cannot optimally use the minerals. To improve their absorption, mineral salts therefore have to be highly diluted (potentized).

Schuessler used the homeopathic potencies D3 (3x), D6 (6x) and D12 (12x) for his therapy. In general, the 6x (dilution 1:1 million) or 12x (1:1 trillion) is taken.

In this naturopathic adviser, I will give you recommendations how to treat and prevent hemorrhoids with Homeopathy, herbal tinctures and Schuessler salts.

I will present you the most proven homeopathic remedies and Schuessler salts, including the appropriate potency and dosage.

Naturopathy works holistically. It does not treat single symptoms only. It treats the whole body, mind and soul.

I wish you much success, joy in life and especially your health.

Robert Kopf

Metabolic blockages in the treatment of hemorrhoids

There are several metabolic blockages which you have to treat for to deacidify and detoxify the body of people suffering from hemorrhoids.

Metabolic blockage No. 1: The acid-base balance

Too much sugar, white flour, meat and sausage acidifies the body. In order to neutralize the acids precious bases are consumed. What is not neutralized, ends up as a "hazardous waste" in the connective tissue and leads to its acidity.

The metabolic process slows down. We get hemorrhoids, gain weight despite calorie conscious diet and exercise.

Metabolic blockage No. 2: The connective tissue

The connective tissue is more than just a connection between the organs. It serves as a nutrient storage and intermediate storage of metabolic products. In the connective tissue the cells dispose their waste products. That the toxins can leave the body, enough mineral salts must be present.

A mineral deficiency causes metabolic residues, acidification and overload with toxins. They remain in the connective tissue and bind water. It comes to hemorrhoids and water retention (edema) in the tissues of the body.

Metabolic blockage No. 3: The digestion

Environmental pollution, lush diet and medication burden the liver, our central metabolic organ. Stomach, pancreas and intestines suffer with.

Many metabolic processes stalled and it comes to hemorrhoids, weight gain, constipation, bloating and stomach problems.

Metabolic blockage No. 4: Our water Resources

Every day the organism produces acids and waste products that have to be filtered out by the kidneys. But part of it also ends up in the connective tissue, because for the removal mineral salts are absent. We get hemorrhoids.

Metabolic blockage No. 5: The protein digestion

Protein is essential for the production of enzymes, hormones, muscles and the connective tissue. However, in the cleavage of proteins ammonia is formed (a strong cytotoxin). The liver converts the ammonia into non-toxic urea, which is excreted in the urine.

Therefore, a high intake of protein is a strong decontamination work for our two kidneys. Hemorrhoids are the result.

Metabolic blockage No. 6: The digestion of fat

We need fats because they provide essential fatty acids. But fat is also the best energy storage in times of need. The body hoards it especially in the thighs and hips, the abdomen and buttocks.

But the adipose tissue is also a deposit for toxins. This stimulates hemorrhoids.

Metabolic blockage No. 7: The carbohydrate digestion

Carbohydrates are energy pure. But in abundance they are also responsible for weight gain and acidification of the body. What is not burned, will be converted and stored in fat. Especially sweets and white flour products are dangerous. They let the blood sugar level rise up rapidly. This leads to a strong insulin release.

Insulin normalizes blood sugar. At the same time burning fat is broken. Insulin leads fats from the meal in the fat stores of the body. In addition, it holds back water in the body and causes rapidly new hunger.

More information for the treatment of your metabolism you will find in my book:

Metabolism, Metabolic syndrome - Treatment with Homeopathy and Schuessler salts

Hemorrhoids - Treatment and prevention with Homeopathy

In addition to your homeopathic treatment of hemorrhoids, you may make a de-acidification health cure of your body with the following recipe:

320 grams of Sodium bicarbonate (Natrium hydrogenkarbonat)
50 grams of Potassium hydrogen carbonate (Kalium hydrogencarbonat)
70 grams of Calcium citrate (Calciumcitrat)
40 grams of Calcium phosphate (Calciumphosphat)
20 grams of Magnesium citrate (Magnesiumcitrat)
Dissolve 1 teaspoon daily at 10 o'clock in the morning (10 am) and at 4 o'clock in the afternoon (4 pm) in 250 ml of lukewarm water. Drink in small sips.

During the day time, in addition to your homeopathic and biochemical treatment, drink 3 cups of tea for the kidneys. In the evening drink one cup of tea for the liver. This will clean the blood and connective tissue and the toxins, acids and metabolic waste products will be extracted quickly.

1) Liver support tea (very important for the treatment of hemorrhoids) and detoxing the body:

Semen Cardui marianae 50.0 (milk thistle), Rhizoma Tormentillae 15.0 (bloodroot), Radix cum Herba Taraxaci 30.0 (dandelion root and herb), Fructi anisidine (anise) 20.0, Fructi Foeniculi (fennel) 20.0, Folia crispae mentha (mint) 15.0
Mix the above listed items together. Add 1 tablespoon into 1 cup (250 ml) cold water and cover for 8 hours. Cook 3 minutes. Let sit covered for 10 minutes and then strain. Drink 1 cup in the evening.

2) Tea for the kidneys and the extraction of metabolic waste and acids through the urinary tract:

Folia Betulae (birch leaves) 30.0, Herba urticae (nettle herb) 30.0, Herba Equiseti (horsetail) 20.0, Herba Virgaureae (goldenrod) 20.0
Mix the above listed ingredients together. Add 2 teaspoons into 1 cup (250 ml) of hot water, let sit covered for 10 minutes. Strain to drink. Drink 3 cups daily.

3) If you suffer from allergies, alternate daily the 2 above mentioned teas with a tea used for the treatment of allergies, to sensitize your body for the treatment of hemorrhoids with Schuessler salts and Homeopathy:

Radix Imperatoriae 20 g, Radix Pimpinellae 20 g, Herba Euphrasiae 10 g, Herba Rutae hortensis 30 g, Rhizoma Graminis 10 g, Herba Absinthii 10 g
Mix the above listed ingredients together. Add 1 teaspoon into 1 cup (250 ml) of water, cook 2 minutes, let sit covered for 10 minutes. Strain to drink. Drink 3 cups daily.

Pay attention to an adequate hydration (water, tea, unsweetened juices).

The kidneys can extract metabolic waste products only if there is enough liquid available. If you exercise a lot, you need more fluid. The water supports the elimination of toxins and waste products of the metabolism. In addition, it prevents hunger.

Drink the most until the afternoon. In the evening drink as little as possible to relieve the bladder.

For enhancing the effect of the homeopathic medicine dissolve the globules in a small glas of water and drink in small sips. Swallow after 1 minute. For stirring please do not use metal spoon.

Do not count the globules in the hand. The manual welding destroys the sprayed drug.

Avoid during the homeopathic treatment the consumption of nicotine, alcohol and spicy foods. They reduce the effectiveness of the sensitive homeopathic remedies.

Abrotanum 3x
Hemorrhoids alternate with rheumatism
Hemorrhoids have a rheumatic cause
Abrotanum strengthens the connective tissue of the hemorrhoids
Increases blood circulation
Opens the small arteries and veins (capillaries)
Depression due to circulatory disorders of the brain.
Abrotanum increases blood circulation in the brain.
Sharp urine
Kidney and bladder diseases
Acne and skin diseases
Abrotanum stimulates the metabolism and the immune system.
3 times a day, take 10 globules, let them melt in your mouth.
Or use Abrotanum tincture: 3 times a day, add 15 drops in some water and drink in small sips.

Absinthium tincture

Hemorrhoids due to metabolic blockages and
environmental toxins.

Strengthens the liver, pancreas, stomach and spleen
(important for the treatment of hemorrhoids).

Anemia and iron defiency

Promotes the formation of blood

Contains iron (important for strong blood vessels)

Immune deficiency

Absinthium strengthens the spleen (important for the
treatment of anemia and immune deficiency)

Strengthen the immune system, extracts environmental
toxins and resolves metabolic blockages.

Gastritis and stomach diseases

Promotes the formation of bile - the intestine is stimulated
by it (70% of our immune system are located in the
intestines). Intestines healthy, man healthy!

Absinthium is a basic remedy for the treatment of
hemorrrhoids and digestive organs.

Proven in the treatment of bloating and flatulence
(meteorism increase the pressure on hemorrhoids).

3 times a day, add 15 drops in some water and drink in
small sips.

Acidum hydrofluoricum 12x

Hemorrhoids
Strengthens the blood vessels and the connective tissue of the hemorrhoids.
Rheumatism - Acidum fluoratum strengthens the articular cartilage.
Skin diseases caused by sunlight.
2 times a day, take 5 globules, let them melt in your mouth.

Acidum muriaticum 4x

Internal hemorrhoids
Anemia and iron deficiency
Acidum muriaticum enhances the absorption of iron in the small intestine.
3 times a day, take 10 globules, let them melt in your mouth.

Acidum nitricum 6x

External hemorrhoids

Stinging and dragging pain in the anus.

Splitter pain in the anal region and stinging pain after defecation.

Cramps during defecation

Cracks (fissures) in the anus

Bloody and mucoid diarrhea

Superficial spider veins and varicose veins

Malodorous flatulence and bloating

Acid regurgitation, sour and bitter taste after eating

Gastritis and peptic ulcer

Heart problems and insomnia

High blood pressure aggravated by stress.

Very nervous and lean people

Life weariness, hopelessness, rejects consolation.

The person catch a cold quickly.

Strong smelling urine

Neurasthenia exacerbated by stress

Overwrought senses

Acidum nitricum strengthens the nerves of people suffering from burnout and neurasthenia, because stress weakens the nerves and immune system.

Acidum nitricum strengthens the immune system and the energy.

The patient has a "band feeling" around the head.

The "Acidum nitricum-Type":

Nervous and slender. The face is dark and looks dried out.

The patient asks for salty and fatty foods.

3 times a day, take 5 globules, let them melt in your mouth.

Acidum phosphoricum 6x

An important metabolic remedy to treat hemorrhoids.
Anemia - Acidum phosphoricum promotes iron absorption in the small intestine.
Normalizes the metabolism and resolves metabolic blockages.
Strengthens the pancreas and the connective tissue of the intestines and hemorrhoids.
Acidum phosphoricum strengthen the nerves and immune system.
The patient is tired and weak.
Loss of concentration, dizziness.
Needs rest and warmth.
3 times a day, take 5 globules, let them melt in your mouth.

Acidum sulph 6x (Acidum sulfuricum D6)

Hemorrhoids of menopausal women due to hormonal changes.
Depression, nervousness and anxiety during menopause.
Heart problems and sleep disorders in the climacteric.
Vomiting, nausea and sweating
Diarrhea and bloating
Celiac disease of women in menopause.
Very helpful for the treatment of gastritis, stomach diseases and a weakened immune system in menopause.
The symptoms are worse at night, in movement and touch.
3 times a day, take 5 globules, let them melt in your mouth.

Aconitum napellus 4x

Acute hemorrhoidal pain

The pain is cutting, ripping and burning with tingling, numbness, redness and heat.

Feeling as if the painful area is swollen.

Worse at night, by dry and cold weather, touch, due to anxiety.

Sensitive to weather changes.

Agony

Afraid to die and delusions.

The person is anxious, nervous, hasty and frightened.

Touch sensitiveness of the belly.

The main symptoms:

Dry and cold winds generate and aggravate the symptoms.

Thirst for cold water.

People with dark hair and dark eyes.

3 times a day, take 10 globules, let them melt in your mouth.

Aesculus tincture

Hemorrhoids

Edema caused by venous circulatory disorders.

Aesculus strengthens the connective tissue of hemorrhoids and veins.

Venous circulatory disorders and venous congestion.

Extracts edema

3 times a day, add 15 drops in some water and drink in small sips.

Agnus castus 3x

Hemorrhoids of women in menopause due to hormonal imbalance.

Immunodeficiency of women in menopause.

Menopausal symptoms

Weather sensitivity, mood swings and depression of women in menopause.

Agnus castus has a regulating effect on the female hormonal system.

3 times a day, take 10 globules, let them melt in your mouth.

Agrimonia eupatoria 3x

Hemorrhoids due to liver weakness and intestinal diseases. Strengthens the stomach, liver, pancreas and intestines (more then 70% of our immune system are located in the intestines).

Bloating and flatulence

Agrimonia promotes the formation of urea and extraction of toxins.

Proven in ascites

Helps to strengthen the defense.

Purifies and detoxifies the body.

3 times a day, take 10 globules, let them melt in your mouth.

Aloe 3x

Hemorrhoids with bloating, slimy diarrhea and rumbling in the abdomen.

Unnoticed departure from winds (flatulence).

Weakness of anal sphincter.

Aloe tonifies the rectum braid.

3 times a day, take 10 globules, let them melt in your mouth.

Alumina 6x

Hemorrhoids

Constipation and bloating

The stool is hard, knotty and slime covered.

The rectum seems paralyzed and has no power to remove the stool.

Even soft stool is extracted difficulty.

No physical discomfort even if for days no bowel movement.

After defecation a feeling as if the rectum would be dragged to the navel.

No feeling of emptiness after defecation.

3 times a day, take 5 globules, let them melt in your mouth.

Ambra 6x

Hemorrhoids due to vegetative disturbances, nervousness, nervous exhaustion and hypersensitivity.

Vascular calcification and circulatory problems

Meteorosensitivity

Depressed mood and vegetative disturbances

Nervousness and nervous exhaustion due to worries

Dysregulation of the autonomic nervous system

Can not unwind in the evening

The person don't like many people around, gets easily upset.

The "Amber" type:

The person is slim, unstable, restless, lean and weak.

Blushes easily

3 times a day, take 5 globules, let them melt in your mouth.

Ammonium carb 12x (Ammonium carbonicum D12)

Hemorrhoids of thick women, panting and gasping for air.

The person is restless, fearful, angry and short of breath.

The person promises much, but does nothing.

Watery and red eyes

Prone Skin

Immunodeficiency

Worsening of the symtoms at night.

2 times a day, take 5 globules, let them melt in your mouth.

Angelica tincture

Hemorrhoids due to a weakness of the digestive organs and environmental toxins.

To strengthen the digestive system and metabolism.

Angelika extracts environmental toxins.

Strengthens the connective tissue of the hemorrhoids and the immune system. The majority of our immune system is located in the abdomen.

Strengthens blood circulation in the abdomen.

Gastritis and stomach diseases

Calms the entire abdomen

Diabetes

Stimulates the blood flow to stomach, pancreas and liver and normalizes the function of the digestive organs.

Intestines healthy, man healthy!

3 times a day, add 15 drops in some water and drink in small sips.

Antimony crudum 4x (Antimonium crudum D4)

Haemorrhoidal knots and lumps

Moist anus

Gastritis and indigestion

Nausea and vomiting

Thick and milky white coating on the tongue.

Diarrhea and constipation alternate

The stool is hard, emptying difficult

Itchy skin in old age

Cold sores

3 times a day, take 10 globules, let them melt in your mouth.

Apis 6x

Inflamed hemorrhoids with stabbing, lancinating, knocking, nagging, pungent pain and burning heat.

Sudden onset of symptoms

Worsening of symptoms at night, by touch and heat.

Relieved by cold applications and in fresh air.

The patient often has edema (fluid retention in the body)

Constipation

The typical Apis patient is apathetic, indifferent, joyless and jealous.

He does not tolerate heat and has no thirst.

3 times a day, take 5 globules, let them melt in your mouth.

Argentum nitricum 6x (Silver nitrate D6)
Acute and painful hemorrhoids
Slimy and bloody diarrhea
He has cramping pain.
For the treatment of hemorrhoids from consumptive people
who are prone to swollen glands, rashes and chronic
diseases.
Too much stomach acid
Also an excellent remedy for the treatment of stomach
ulcers.
The face is dark and has a dried-up appearance.
The person is always in a hurry, hectic and restless.
He believes the time passes by too slowly.
The "silver nitrate patient" demands for sweets and sugar
but he can not tolerate.
He also like to have salt and cool fresh air.
The patient suffers from anxiety, haste and bloating.
Argentum nitricum strengthens the immune system of
consumptive people.
The person catch quickly a cold.
Modalities:
Exacerbation of pain in heat
Improvement by strong pressure
Associated symptoms:
Splitter feeling in the painful areas
The pain:
Drilling and cutting
Coming suddenly and disappearing suddenly
Sometimes the pain starts with sunrise and stops with
sunset.
3 times a day, take 5 globules, let them melt in your mouth.

Arnica tincture

Hemorrhoidal pain due to abdominal pressure.
Stimulates the healing processes of the inflammed hemorrhoids.
Arnica promotes blood circulation and strengthens the blood vessels.
The Arnica patient perceives his body sore and bruised, the bed is too hard.
The patient is afraid of contact with other people.
Arnica is the main remedy for arterial and venous circulatory disorders. As a result, the body is better supplied with oxygen and nutrients and the metabolism will be strengthened.
A strange symptom:
He pretends to be healthy, even if he is sick.
The modalities:
Aggravation of hemorrhoidal pain in movement
Improvement by rest
Diseases of the blood vessels
3 times a day, add 15 drops in some water and drink in small sips.

Arsenicum album 6x

Hemorrhoids with burning pain, swelling and inflamation.
The pain usually occurs at the same time.
Aggravation at midnight. His worst time is between 12
clock at midnight and 2 clock in the morning (2 am).
The intake of Arsenicum album between 6 clock (6 pm)
and 7 clock in the evening (7 pm) often prevent the
nocturnal pain attack.
Desire for fresh air, despite feeling cold.
Great restlessness, anxiety and fatigue. Want always to
move.
Loathing of food
Different colored and smelly feces
Helps very well in a large fluid loss due to diarrhea and
vomiting.
The patient is sensitive to cold, choosy and frightened.
A broken and emaciated person with a weak immune
system.
Cold, dull and blemished skin, sunken face with hollow
eyes.
The skin is waxy, dry and flaky.
The secretions are corrosive, excoriating, watery and
burning.
Polyuria (frequent urination with a lot of urine) and great
thirst.
Melancholy, despair, indifference, depression and anxiety.
The person is exhausted, pale, emaciated, frightened and
tired of life.
Fear of death and sorrow
Suicidal thoughts without fear
Nervous itching
The abdomen is sensitive to pressure.
Circulatory problems
3 times a day, take 5 globules, let them melt in your mouth.

Asafoetida 4x

Hemorrhoids due to nervous disorders of the digestive organs.
Bloating
Popping burps and smelly winds
3 times a day, take 10 globules, let them melt in your mouth.

Aurum metallicum 6x

Hemorrhoids of the red-cheeked and obese people.
The main remedy for all venous problems (hemorrhoids are veins).
Suppuration and inflammation of hemorrhoids and intestinal mucosa.
Circulatory problems due to high blood pressure (hypertension).
High blood pressure and red face.
Edema caused by metabolic blockade.
Strengthens the immune system and eliminates metabolic blockages.
Induration of glandular organs
An obese person with immunodeficiency, cardiac insufficiency and angina pectoris.
Sclerosis of the brain. The person will be increasingly depressed, irritable and jaded.
Decline in memory
A grumpy patient.
Hopeless blackness. He talks about death.
Aurum metallicum supports weight loss and increases well-being.
The main symptoms:
Worries about the future, even if he's okay.
Always takes everything very seriously.

The accompanying symptoms:
Great sensitivity to cold.
3 times a day, take 5 globules, let them melt in your mouth.

Barium iodatum 6x (Barium jodatum D6)
Hemorrhoids due to obesity and a slow metabolism.
Obesity because of an underactive thyroid gland (this causes a slow metabolism).
Immunodeficiency due to an underactive thyroid (slow metabolism).
Strengthens the immune system
Stimulates the brain metabolism
For the prevention of arteriosclerosis and cancer.
Barium iodatum strengthens the thyroid. This stimulates the metabolism and increases the temperature of the body. This in turn strengthens the immune system. Pathogens and cancer cells are highly susceptible to increased body temperature.
Stimulates the arterial blood flow too. Thus, the hemorrhoids and body cells are better supplied with oxygen and nutrients.
3 times a day, take 5 globules, let them melt in your mouth.

Belladonna 6x

Hemorrhoids

The character of pain is raging, burning, lancinating, violent, sudden, throbbing and of short duration.

Sudden onset of the symptoms and sudden termination.

Black before his eyes.

Modalities:

Hypersensitivity of the senses to light, noise, vibration and odors.

Worse from noise, touch, vibration and cold.

Improvement in a warm room, with heat in general and at rest.

Significantly, inflammatory pain of Belladonna is always accompanied by a local heat. This is also noticeable with the palpating (scanning) hand. Nevertheless, the patient wants to be wrapped up warm. Cold worsen his condition.

The Belladonna patient requests in fever lemons, is hot, red and tends to delirium (confusion).

He has no thirst.

3 times a day, take 5 globules, let them melt in your mouth.

Berberis 3x

Hemorrhoids have a rheumatic cause.

Acidification of the body

Articular gout, rheumatism

Berberis stimulates liver, pancreas and kidneys.

Diseases of the pancreas, liver and gallbladder.

Irritable bowel syndrome with watery diarrhea.

Shooting and cramping hemorrhoidal pain radiating from one point.

Spasmodic pain can be facilitated by Berberis.

Diabetes

3 times a day, take 10 globules, let them melt in your mouth.

Bothrops 6x

To relieve the hemorrhoidal pain.

3 times a day, take 5 globules, let them melt in your mouth.

Bursa pastoris tincture

Hemorhoids

Strengthens the blood vessels and stops bleeding.

3 times a day, add 15 drops in some water and drink in small sips.

Calabar 4x

Hemorrhoids due to obesity
Strengthens the metabolism of liver and pancreas for to lose weight.
Stimulates digestion and metabolism of the body.
3 times a day, take 10 globules, let them melt in your mouth.

Calcarea 12x (Calcium carbonicum D12)

An important remedy of "lymphatic constitution" for the treatment of hemorrhoids.
Neurasthenia, nervous weakness and depression.
The patient is gloomy, moody and indifferent.
A fearful and hesitant person.
Immune deficiency and metabolic disorders.
Rashes and frequent colds
Sour sweat after the slightest exertion on the head and neck.
Strong foot perspiration
Persistent bloating and constipation
The stool seems like lime.
The feces smell like rotten eggs.
Regurgitation and vomiting
The patient feels better during constipation.
The modalities:
Aggravation of symptoms by cold and damp weather, during full moon.
Improvement by heat and drought.
2 times a day, take 5 globules, let them melt in your mouth.

Calendula tincture

Hemorrhoids
A very good wound healing remedy.
Eliminates inflammations
Invigorating the blood vessels and lymph vessels.
Strengthens the lymphatic system (important for a strong immune system and to treat hemorrhoids).
Increases the metabolic function.
Purifies the blood.
3 times a day, add 15 drops in some water and drink in small sips.

Cantharis 6x

Acute hemorrhoidal pain
The pain is like from a knife, cramping, drilling, cutting, radiating in different directions and burning.
Thirst, but with aversion to all fluids.
3 times a day, take 5 globules, let them melt in your mouth.

Capsicum 6x

Burning hemorrhoids and mucous membranes with swelling.
Modalities:
Worse by the slightest touch and vibration.
The pain:
Burning and stinging, as if sprinkled with pepper.
General chilliness
3 times a day, take 5 globules, let them melt in your mouth.

Carbo vegetabilis 12x

Hemorrhoids in old age

Great weakness, exhaustion, fatigue, lack of air and faint inclination

The remedy of age besides Barium carb (Barium carbonicum).

Depression in old age

Poor general condition, especially in old age.

Strong desire for fresh air and coolness despite chilliness.

Spasmodic cough with shortness of breath and blue tarnished face.

Burning sensation in the chest

Bubbling and whistling sounds when breathing.

Poorly soluble and viscous sputum

Carbo vegetabilis strengthens the defense force of the elderly.

The modalities:

Worsening of symptoms at night and from warmth.

Improvement by fresh air.

2 times a day, take 5 globules, let them melt in your mouth.

Cardui benedikti 3x

Hemorrhoids due to weakness of the liver.

Strengthens pancreas and liver.

Edema and hemorrhoids due to liver insufficiency.

Stimulates bile flow

Bloating

3 times a day, take 10 globules, let them melt in your mouth.

Carduus marianus tincture

Hemorrhoids due to liver and gall bladder diseases.
Strengthens the pancreas and liver.
Supports the metabolism from pancreas and liver.
3 times a day, add 15 drops in a small glass of water and drink in small sips.

Centaurium tincture

Hemorrhoids due to a weak connective tissue and a weakness of the digestive organs.
Anemia and iron deficiency
Promotes the formation of blood
Contains iron
Strengthens the spleen (important for the treatment of hemorrhoids and anemia)
Promotes iron absorption in the small intestine. Iron is important for strong blood vessels.
Irritable bowel syndrome
3 times a day, add 15 drops in a small glass of water and drink in small sips.

Ceonothus 3x

If hemorrhoidal pain is related to the spleen, for example after splenectomy or a disease of the spleen.
Hemorrhoids after gonorrhea
The patient can not lay on his left side.
Dirty and yellowish coated tongue
Anemia
3 times a day, take 10 globules, let them melt in your mouth.

Chamomilla 4x

Hemorrhoids

Flatulence and cramping abdominal pain

The stools are differently colored, look like chopped eggs and have a sour or putrid smell.

Particularly suitable for children with abdominal pain, moodiness and restlessness.

Feverish infections with great sensitivity to pain.

Gastritis and vomiting due to anger.

Eczema and dermatitis of the children with itching.

The patient is moody and stubborn, hypersensitive and restless.

The hemorrhoidal pain is worse by heat, while thinking of the complaints, mental exertion, hot drinks and drafts.

Associated symptoms:

The painful areas are usually hot and flushed.

Tearing and drawing hemorrhoidal pain, like from electric shocks.

Mostly left-sided complaints

Numbness, also alternating with pain.

Remark: The reaction of the patient is not always proportionate to the pain, because the "Chamomilla Type" is very sensitive to pain.

3 times a day, take 10 globules, let them melt in your mouth.

Chelidonium 6x

Hemorrhoids with itching due to liver and gall bladder diseases.
Strengthens the function of pancreatic tissue and liver.
Relaxes the bile ducts.
Feces as from a sheep.
Chelidonium extracts metabolic waste.
3 times a day, take 5 globules, let them melt in your mouth.

Chimaphila 6x

Acute inflammation of the hemorrhoids.
Feeling of swelling in the anal region (as if sitting on a ball).
3 times a day, take 5 globules, let them melt in your mouth.

China tincture

Hemorrhoids with bleeding

Intestinal mucosal bleeding

China strengthens the metabolism, immune system, pancreas and liver.

Bitter taste, yellowish coated tongue.

Abdominal pressure, bloating, diarrhea, nausea and vomiting.

General fatigue and exhaustion

Eczema and dermatitis

Frequent common colds and attacks of fever.

Gout, rheumatism and nerve pain

Usually the left side of the body is affected.

Great sensitiveness of the affected areas to touch but improvement by firm pressure.

Circulatory problems, meteorosensitivity and neurasthenia.

Anemia

Insomnia due to flood of thoughts.

Physical and emotional hypersensitivity.

General weakness and debility

He does not tolerate fruit or milk.

Worsening of symptoms with a light touch, drafts, cold and after the loss of body fluids.

Man is never really healthy.

Subfebrile body temperature (mild fever, often after antibiotic treatment).

Modalities:

Periodic pain at certain times of day.

Improvement by firm pressure and fresh air.

Accompanying symptom: Painful hair

3 times a day, add 15 drops in a small glass of water and drink in small sips.

Cichorium tincture
Hemorrhoids due to weakness of pancreas and liver.
Strengthens the connective tisse of the hemorrhoids.
Irritable bowel syndrome
Strengthens liver and pancreas
Promotes bile formation to reduce cholesterol levels
Diabetes
3 times a day, add 15 drops in a small glass of water and drink in small sips.

Cicuta virosa 3x
Hemorrhoids with stinging pain.
3 times a day, take 10 globules, let them melt in your mouth.

Cimicifuga 12x
Hemorrhoids of women due to hormonal imbalance and menopause.
Cimicifuga regulates the female hormonal balance.
Depression, nervous agitation, insomnia and anxiety.
Spurious heart pain (the heart is healthy despite complaints).
Pain in the abdomen and chest
Hot flashes, nervous agitation
Defense weakness of women due to hormonal imbalances and menopause.
Restlessness, fear, hysteria and delusions.
A mistrustful person
2 times a day, take 5 globules, let them melt in your mouth.

Cistus canadensis 3x

Itchy hemorrhoids and mucous membranes.

Proven in cold sore with itchy blisters.

Itchy skin diseases

Inflammation of the lymphatic glands

3 times a day, take 10 globules. Let them melt in your mouth.

Cochlearia tincture

Hemorrhoids due to a weakness of the spleen.

Anemia and iron deficiency

Promotes the formation of blood

Contains iron

Strengthens the spleen (important for the treatment of hemorrhoids and anemia)

3 times a day, add 15 drops in a small glass of water and drink in small sips.

Colchicum 4x

Hemorrhoids due to gout and rheumatism.

Joint pain

Modalities:

Worse by cold, before and during a change of weather, wet conditions, at night, from sunset to sunrise. Worse are the symptoms also due to food smells and touch.

Improvement by heat and bed rest.

Associated symptoms:

Vibration of the muscles

Edematous swelling of the affected body region.

Twitches and spasms

The pain:

Tearing and wandering around.

Rheumatic pain especially on the left side of the body.

Keynotes:

General fatigue, inner cold

Vomiting and nausea due to food odors.

3 times a day, take 10 globules. Let them melt in your mouth.

Collinsonia 4x

Hemorrhoids

Chronic bleeding and painful hemorrhoids

Feeling of chopsticks, sand or gravel in the rectum.

Obstinate constipation with colic

3 times a day, take 10 globules. Let them melt in your mouth.

Colocynth 6x (Clocynthis D6)

Hemorrhoids with swelling and spasmodic pain, as by an iron clamp.

The pain:

Like lightning, cramping, burning and stinging.

Modalities:

Worse by anger, movement, disgust and fear.

Light pressure, touch and warmth are unbearable.

Improvement by rest and strong pressure.

The accompanying symptoms:

Numbness, restlessness, shivering

3 times a day, take 5 globules. Let them melt in your mouth.

Condurango tincture

Hemorrhoids due to liver weakness

Constipation

Stimulates the liver, pancreas and digestive glands.

3 times a day, add 15 drops in a small glass of water and drink in small sips.

Crataegus tincture (hawthorn)
Hemorrhoids due to cardiac insufficiency.
Disturbance of blood pressure
Arrhythmias and angina pectoris
Circulatory problems and nervous heart
Promotes blood circulation in the heart
A perfect remedy for heart care - Crataegus prevents calcification of the coronary vessels.
3 times a day, add 15 drops in a small glass of water and drink in small sips.

Cynara scolymus tincture
Hemorrhoids due to insufficient pancreas- and liver function.
Stimulates the pancreas, liver and gall bladder system.
Strengthens the liver and assists in detoxification of the body.
An excellent protection for liver and pancreas.
3 times a day, add 15 drops in a small glass of water and drink in small sips.

Dolichos pruriens 3x
Hemorrhoids with itching due to a liver disease.
Itching skin diseases caused by liver disease.
3 times a day, take 10 globules, let them melt in your mouth.

Equisetum tincture

Hemorrhoids due to a weak connective tissue of the blood vessels and an acidification of the body.

Strengthens blood vessels and connective tissue of the hemorrhoids.

Contains silica (important for the treatment of hemorrhoids)

Equisetum purifies the urinary tract.

3 times a day, add 15 drops in a small glass of water and drink in small sips.

Erigeron canadensis 3x

Bleeding hemorrhoids and intestinal mucosa

3 times a day, take 10 globules. Let them melt in your mouth.

Fucus vesiculosus 4x

Hemorrhoids due to a weak thyroid and slow metabolism.

Stimulates the thyroid gland, metabolism and digestion.

Do not take if an overactive thyroid.

3 times a day, take 10 globules, let them melt in your mouth.

Fumaria tincture

Hemorrhoids due to a weak liver and slow metabolism.

Fumaria stimulates the whole metabolism of the body.

3 times a day, add 15 drops in a small glass of water and drink in small sips.

Glechoma hederacea tincture

Hemorrhoids due to anemia and iron deficiency.
Promotes the formation of blood.
Contains iron
Strengthens the spleen (important for the treatment of anemia and hemorrhoids)
Promotes iron absorption in the small intestine. Iron is important for strong blood vessels.
3 times a day, add 15 drops in a small glass of water and drink in small sips.

Graphites 6x

Hemorrhoids due to intestinal disorders and obesity.
Hemorrhoids from people who are more passive in their behaviour and their metabolism works slowly.
Tendency to skin problems and colds.
The skin is itchy, sore, mostly dry, scabby, yellow and pale.
Blackheads, acne.
Skin disorders with sticky secretions.
Smelling foot sweat and stinking night sweats.
A proven remedy for the treatment of hemorrhoids, chronic skin diseases, metabolic disorders and immune deficiency.
Improvement by hot food and drinks.
3 times a day, take 5 globules, let them melt in your mouth.

Hamamelis virginica tincture

Hemorrhoids with bleeding

Bleeding of the intestinal mucosa

Hemorrhoids caused by venous congestions.

Strengthens and tones the veins and hemorrhoids.

Varicose veins

Rashes of the skin

Strengthens and tones the veins and the connective tissue of the hemorrhoids.

3 times a day, add 15 drops in a small glass of water and drink in small sips.

Helleborus niger 3x

Hemorrhoids due to a weakness of the kidneys and heart.

Helleborus strengthens the heart muscle.

Stimulates the metabolism from the kidneys. This relieves the blood vessels and is important for the treatment of hemorrhoids.

Extracts metabolic waste and acid.

An intact renal function strengthens the immune system.

Skin diseases due to weak kidneys.

Note: Skin and kidneys are from the perspective of naturopathy siblings. Kidneys healthy, skin healthy

3 times a day, take 10 globules, let them melt in your mouth.

Helonias dioica 3x

Hemorrhoids of women with a weak connective tissue.
Helonias strengthens the connective tissue of the
hemorrhoids.
Uterine prolapse
3 times a day, take 10 globules, let them melt in your
mouth.

Hydrastis 4x

Hemorrhoids, phlebitis and varicose veins.
3 times a day, take 10 globules, let them melt in your
mouth.

Hypericum tincture

Hemorrhoids due to psychological problems and
depression.
A classic remedy for mental illness.
Depression, nervousness and irritability.
Affects mood enhancing and vegetative balancing.
Strengthens the liver.
3 times a day, add 15 drops in a small glass of water and
drink in small sips.

Juglans cinerea 4x

Hemorrhoids due to obesity with high cholesterol level and hyperlipidemia.

Disorders of pancreas and liver function.

Promotes bile formation. This supports fat metabolism.

Stimulates the liver in cholesterol reduction and strengthens the pancreas in digestive functions.

3 times a day, take 10 globules, let them melt in your mouth.

Juniperus tincture

Hemorrhoids due to weak kidneys and an acidification of the body.

Strengthens the kidneys and stomach.

Promotes the formation of blood

Contains iron. This is important for a healthy skin.

Purifying the organism and enhancing the immune system.

Do not use in an acute kidney disease. Juniper is highly stimulating the kidneys.

2 times a day, add 10 drops in a small glass of water. Drink in small sips.

Levisticum tincture
Hemorrhoids due to cardiac and renal weakness.
Edema
Promotes the blood circulation of the urogenital tract.
Strengthens the kidneys and heart muscles
An aphrodisiac
3 times a day, add 15 drops in a small glass of water and drink in small sips.

Lilium tigrinum 3x
Hemorrhoids of women in menopause
Women with menopausal symptoms, heart problems and circulatory problems.
Incontinence and complaints by uterine prolapse in menopause.
Irritable mood states
Invigorates and strengthens the blood vessel and walls of the hemorrhoids.
3 times a day, take 10 globules, let them melt in your mouth.

Lithium carb 4x (Lithium carbonicum D4)
Hemorrhoids due to gout and rheumatic diseases.
Uric acid in the blood
3 times a day, take 10 globules, let them melt in your mouth.

Lycopodium 6x

Hemorrhoids

The pain is chronic and burning.

Disorders of pancreas and liver function

Inflammation and disorders of the hepatobiliary system.

Swelling of the liver, obstinate constipation.

Flatulence and bloating even after eating small amounts.

Cravings, but saturated after little food.

Lycopodium stops the nightly cravings and cravings for sweets.

Sour vomiting

Flatulence and rumbling in the abdomen.

The stool is difficult to excrete, hard and sparse.

No empty feeling after a bowel movement.

Much gas formation in the stomach, a loud rumbling and gurgling in the bowels.

Heartburn and great fatigue after eating.

Constant burping

Feeling of helplessness

Complaints mostly on the right side of the body.

The typical "Lycopodium type" requires sweets, sugar and hot drinks.

He is nasty on awakening, but otherwise the symptoms are better in the morning.

Irascibility, brooks no contradiction.

Kidney stones

Red gries (such as brick dust sediment) in the urine.

The "Lycopodium patient" has two strange symptoms:

"He weeps, if somebody would like to thank him" and "one foot is warm, the other foot is cold".

The modalities:

Aggravation of symptoms between 16 clock in the afternoon and 20 clock in the evening, through heat, touch, anger and tight clothing.

Improvement by belching, by hot food and drinks, exercise and cold air.

3 times a day, take 5 globules, let them melt in your mouth.

Madar 4x

Hemorrhoids caused by obesity

Madar affects the hunger center in the brain and curbs the appetite.

Detoxifying the organism

3 times a day, take 10 globules, let them melt in your mouth.

Melilotus tincture

Hemorrhoids

Strengthens the connective tissue of the hemorrhoids.

Venous circulation disorders

Weakness of the veins and lymphatic vessels. Strengthens veins and lymphatic vessels.

Melilotus improves blood and lymph flow.

Thins the blood

High blood pressure

Heavy rush of blood to the head.

Red face

Improvement through nosebleeds

Migraine and headache

Strengthens the immune system and supports the metabolism.

Extracts metabolic waste and toxins.

3 times a day, add 15 drops in a small glass of water and drink in small sips.

Mercurius corossivus 4x

Painful hemorrhoids caused by degenerative blood vessels.
The skin is cold, pale and dripping with sweat.
Salivation with salty taste
Weakness of memory
Tenesmus (violent and painful urination) with a strong burning sensation in the urethra.
3 times a day, take 10 globules, let them melt in your mouth.

Mercurius solubilis 4x

Inflammation and swelling of the hemorrhoids.
Hemorrhoids with tearing, stinging and nagging pain especially at night.
Modalities:
Worse by heat, warmth of bed, touch, damp and rainy weather, at night, by drafts.
Improvement by rest.
3 times a day, take 10 globules, let them melt in your mouth.

Millefolium tincture

Hemorrhoids caused by weak blood vessels.
Stops bleeding and inflammation
Strengthens the connective tissue of the hemorrhoids.
High blood pressure
Millefolium regulates the blood pressure
Edema and hypertension caused by weak blood vessels.
Promotes blood circulation and strengthens the blood
vessels. As a result, the body is better supplied with oxygen
and nutrients and the metabolism will be strengthened.
Anemia and iron deficiency
Promotes the formation of blood
Contains iron. This is very important for healthy and strong
hemorrhoids.
Strengthens the spleen (important for the treatment of
anemia and hemorrhoids)
Promotes iron absorption in the small intestine.
For the prevention of cancer.
Millefolium strengthens the immune system.
Relaxes and calms the abdomen.
Promotes the circulation of the digestive organs.
Bloating
3 times a day, add 15 drops in a small glass of water and
drink in small sips.

Myrrhis odorata 3x

Internal and external hemorrhoids.
Strengthens the connective tissue of the hemorrhoids.
3 times a day, take 10 globules, let them melt in your
mouth.

Nux vomica 6x

Hemorrhoids of the "managers"

Feeling as if a nail is in the anus.

Bright blood is discharged with the stool.

Hemorrhoids as a consequence of alcohol abuse, coffee, overeating and long nights.

High blood pressure due to stress and anger.

Hemorrhoids, overwrought nerves, nausea and vomiting of drunkards.

Circulatory problems with vertigo, especially after stimulant abuse (alcohol, nicotine).

A feeling of constriction

Tendency to convulsions and periodic complaints.

Diseases of the pancreas due to alcohol abuse.

Tearing, stinging and contractive pain in the abdomen.

Swelling of the liver

Gallstones

Inflammation of the bile ducts.

Large and hard stools. Always has the feeling that the evacuation would be incomplete.

Frequent need for toileting, but without success.

Feeling as if a stone in the stomach.

Frequent belching of sour or bitter liquid.

Fever

The "Nux vomica type":

Irritable, choleric, nervous, lively, emaciated.

He considers himself to be very important.

The Modalities:

Worse are the symptoms after midnight, in the early morning, by cold and dry weather, after drinking wine and coffee.

Improvement in wet weather, in warm rooms.

The pain:

Tearing, astringent, cramping, dull.

3 times a day, take 5 globules, let them melt in your mouth.

Okoubaka

Hemorrhoids due to environmental toxins.

Toxins, for example food additives and environmental toxins, block the metabolism, can cause hemorrhoids and chronic diseases.

Okoubaka detoxifies the body, eliminates metabolic waste and environmental toxins. Strengthens the immune system. Very helpful for the treatment of indigestion after eating spoiled food, meat and fat.

For thorough detoxification, elimination and extraction of environmental toxins and other residues, please make the following treatment. In addition, please drink the above mentioned teas.

1st to 4th week:
Okoubaka 3x
3 times a day, take 10 globules, let them melt in your mouth.

5th to 8th week:
Okoubaka 4x
3 times a day, take 10 globules, let them melt in your mouth.

9th to 12th week:
Okoubaka 6x
3 times a day, take 5 globules, let them melt in your mouth.

13th to 16th week:
Okoubaka 12x
2 times a day, take 5 globules, let them melt in your mouth.

Then a further 3 months:
Okoubaka 30x
1 time a week, take 5 globules, let them melt in your mouth.

Paeonia 3x

Very successful in the treatment of hemorrhoids.
3 times a day, take 10 globules, let them melt in your mouth.

Passiflora tincture

Hemorrhoids due to nervousness, neurasthenia and stress.
Nervous heart
Sleeplessness
3 times a day, add 15 drops in a small glass of water and drink in small sips.

Phaseolum tincture

Hemorrhoids due to an acidification of the body.
Cleans and de-acidifies the connective tissue and the whole body.
The main remedy for stimulating diuresis.
Proven in high uric acid and ascites (abdominal dropsy).
3 times a day, add 15 drops in a small glass of water and drink in small sips.

Phosphorus amorphus 6x

Inflamed, bleeding and itchy hemorrhoids.

Phosphorus is an important metabolic remedy.

Phosphorus strengthens the function of liver, pancreas and immune system.

Nervousness, hectic red spots on the face. A slender and frosty person.

Depression and self-pity. Labile moods, he likes to be comforted.

Phosphorus is known in naturopathy as a "light bringer".

He is afraid of darkness, aloneness and thunderstorms.

Quickly furious. The patient reacts violently to everything and is exhausted quickly.

Night sweats

Keynotes: Scary, especially at dusk.

He is slim, tall, blonde and has fine hair.

Bleed easily

The accompanying symptoms:

Craving for salt, cold drinks or ice cream.

Get bruises easily and is very sensitive to pain.

In rapid movements (turning the head) he get dizzy.

3 times a day, take 5 globules, let them melt in your mouth.

Podophyllum 6x

Hemorrhoids due to obesity
Constipation (causes hemorrhoids)
An important remedy for the treatment of obesity and hemorrhoids.
Disorders of the hepatobiliary system
Podophyllum stimulates the formation of juices in the pancreas and liver.
Gastritis and stomach ulcer
Empty feeling in the stomach
Morning sickness with vomiting
Nausea and dizziness
3 times a day, take 5 globules, let them melt in your mouth.

Psorinum 12x

Hemorrhoids due to persistent metabolic disorders.

The typical "Psorinum patient" is frosty, cautious, afraid to wash and has an unpleasant perspiration.

Desperate anxiety

Chronic eczema and dermatitis

Obstinate and itchy skin conditions

The skin is dry, pale and yellow.

Stinking foot sweat and stinking night sweats.

Lichen, scabs, acne and blackheads.

The modalities:

Aggravation of symptoms from cold, sun, wind, and when changing from warm to cold weather.

Improvement at rest, when lying down and through eating.

Striking well-being on the day before an attack.

2 times a day, take 5 globules, let them melt in your mouth.

Pulsatilla 6x

Hemorrhoids

Constipation after fat and a lot of food.

Diarrhea and constipation alternating.

Inflammation and disorders of the female reproductive organs.

Worse in a warmth, especially in warm rooms.

The "Pulsatilla Type" is moody, sensitive and whiny, loves compassion.

Chilliness, lack of appetite and without thirst.

Neurasthenia and hypersensitivity to noise.

Self-pity

Moody, wants comfort, gentle, melancholy and anxious.

Has fear of death and is afraid of people.

Keynotes:

Soft and gentle disposition, shy, timid, tearful, chilly, anemic.

3 times a day, take 5 globules, let them melt in your mouth.

Quassia amara tincture

Hemorrhoids due to a weakness of pancreas and liver.
Cleanses the body fluids and stimulates the liver,
gallbladder and pancreas.
Meteorism (bloating causes hemorrhoids)
An important metabolic remedy
Strengthens the immune system
Frontal headache (often a sign of liver dysfunction).
3 times a day, add 15 drops in a small glass of water and
drink in small sips.

Rhizoma Helenii tincture

Hemorrhoids due to metabolic disorders.
An excellent metabolic remedy.
Strengthens and regenerates pancreas and liver.
Stimulates the connective tissue and immune system.
For the prevention of cancer.
Diabetes
3 times a day, add 15 drops in a small glass of water and
drink in small sips.

Ruta graveolens 4x

Inflamed and swollen hemorrhoids

Proven in hemorrhoidal pain

Ruta strengthens the connective tissue of the hemorrhoids.

Stimulates blood circulation

Complains due to circulatory disorders and rheumatism.

Muscle pain caused by overexertion

Inflamed muscles, ligaments and tendons

Tendovaginitis

In the morning the pain is worse.

Periosteum injuries

Worse by lying down

The pain seems to come out from the bones.

The patient has to walk around to ease his pain.

3 times a day, take 10 globules, let them melt in your mouth.

Sepia 12x

Hemorrhoids of women

Feeling of heaviness in the rectum.

No relief after defecation

Pain in the rectum during defecation and long time after stool.

The stool is hard, knotty, too little, covered with blood and mucus.

Menopausal symptoms with headache, sleeplessness, nervousness, depression and anxiety.

The woman sighs, moans and smiles alternately.

Dropping of the eyelids

Bleedings in menopause

Multiple disorders of the female reproductive organs.

Sad and cries often without knowing why.

The "Sepia type" has a yellowish complexion, hates compassion and wants to be left alone.

Mentally sluggish and irritable

Rapid change of mood

Indifferent to obligations

The stomach feels empty and desolate.

The hepatic region is painful and stinging.

Brown spots on the skin of the abdomen.

Diarrhea after milk consumption.

2 times a day, take 5 globules, let them melt in your mouth.

Solidago tincture

Hemorrhoids due to a weakness of the kidneys and an acidification of the body.

To stimulate the kidneys, blood cleansing, deacidification and extraction of toxins via the kidneys.

Solidago works diuretic and extracts edema.

The kidneys always must be treated as well from the perspective of natural medicine for the treatment of hemorrhoids.

Skin diseases - kidneys and skin are from the perspective of naturopathy siblings. In case of skin problems a remedy for the kidney must therefore always be used.

3 times a day, add 15 drops in a small glass of water and drink in small sips.

Spigelia 6x

Increase and decrease of hemorrhoidal pain with the movement of the sun.

The Pain:

Violent, lancinating, spasmodic

Worse from motion, touch, vibration, weather changes and by stooping.

Improvement by constant pressure.

Associated symptoms:

Heart anxiety, heart stitches and tightness in the chest.

Fear of sharp objects.

Shivering and chills all over the body.

3 times a day, take 5 globules, let them melt in your mouth.

Spongia 4x

Hemorrhoids due to an underactive thyroid.

Spongia stimulates the thyroid gland.

The immune system and metabolism are strengthened.

3 times a day, take 10 globules, let them melt in your mouth.

Staphysagria 6x

Hemorrhoids

Strengthens the connective tissue of the hemorrhoids.

Staphysagria has a strengthening effect on the anal sphincter.

Good for sphincter muscles that were stretched by surgery.

Staphysagria is a great remedy for suppressed anger and repressed emotions.

Agitation of mind and nervous system.

Great indignation about things that were done by others or himself.

Keynotes:

Sensitive to what others think about him.

Deep-set eyes with blue edges as after a night of drinking.

Modalities:

Worse at night, by anger and indignation.

Improvement of the symptoms after breakfast, by heat and bed rest.

3 times a day, take 5 globules, let them melt in your mouth.

Sulphur 12x

Hemorrhoids due to a reduced metabolism.

Itching and burning at night.

Sulfur is an important catalyst to regenerate a sluggish and blocked metabolism.

The skin looks gray, dirty and wrinkled.

Stinking flatulence in the morning.

Stool with a feeling as if something remained.

The stool is hard, as if burnt, large and painful.

The stool is held back because of the pain when emptying.

Hunger at 11 clock in the morning.

Appetite for everything, especially on fat.

Pushes away the cover at night, stretching his legs out of bed.

Redness of the orifices

Sharp and excoriating secretions.

Sulfur strengthens the immune system and regenerates the pancreas and liver.

Sulfur is an important catalyst to bring a stalled metabolism and immune system back on track.

Chronic diseases

Sulfur is detoxifying the body.

2 times a day, take 5 globules, let them melt in your mouth.

Symphytum tincture

Hemorrhoids

Strengthens the blood vessels and the connective tissue of the hemorrhoids.

Stimulates the metabolism of the blood vessels.

Promotes hepatic blood flow and is important for the small intestine.

Anemia and iron deficiency

Promotes the formation of blood

Contains iron (important for blood vessels) and vitamin B12

Strengthens the spleen (important for the treatment of anemia and hemorrhoids)

Promotes iron absorption in the small intestine.

Strengthens the metabolism of the bones (important for blood formation and an intact immune system).

Rheumatism - the rheumatic pain emanates from the bone.

3 times a day, add 15 drops in a small glass of water and drink in small sips.

Taraxacum tincture

Hemorrhoids due to a weakness of the liver and an acidification of the body.

Strengthens the liver-bile system, pancreas and kidneys.

Detoxifies the connective tissue, organism and acts cholagogue.

Strengthens the immune system

Cleans the blood and stimulates the metabolism.

Nausea due to a weakness of pancreas and liver.

Eczema and skin diseases

3 times a day, add 15 drops in a small glass of water and drink in small sips.

Thuja 6x

Hemorrhoidal pain after vaccination

Immune deficiency after vaccination

Thuja extracts toxins and strengthens the immune system.

The modalities:

Worse by cold, wet weather, change of weather, storm and tempest, after drinking tea and eating onions.

Improvement by heat, warm applications and re-emerging sweat.

The complaints are worse at 3 clock in the morning and 15 clock in the afternoon.

3 times a day, take 5 globules, let them melt in your mouth.

Urtica urens tincture

Hemorrhoides due to an acidification of the body and metabolic weakness.

Allergic, itchy and inflamed skin rash with small pimples and blisters.

Cold sores with itching

Skin conditions with blisters

Diuretic - stimulates kidneys and metabolism.

Urtica detoxifies and de-acidifies the body.

3 times a day, add 15 drops in a small glass of water and drink in small sips.

Zinkum valerianicum 12x

Hemorrhoids due to nervousness and neurasthenia.

The person is restless and has a restlessness in the legs (restless legs).

Poor sleep

Twitching in bed, like electric shocks.

2 times a day, take 5 globules, let them melt in your mouth.

A homeopathic prescription for the treatment of hemorrhoids and for stimulating the metabolism:
Helianthus tuberosus 3x dil., Duboisia 3x dil., Euphorbia cyparissias 3x dil. aa 10.0, Extractum Fucus vesiculosus (if not overactive thyroid occurs), Extractum Frangulae (buckthorn bark), Extractum Alchemilla (Lady's Mantle) aa 15.0
3 times a day, add 15 drops in a small glass of water and drink in small sips before eating.

A recipe to treat hemorrhoids and for strengthening the pancreas, liver and bile:
Cardui marianae tincture, Cardui benedikti tincture aa 25.0, China tincture, Chelidonium 6x aa 10.0, Flor de Piedra 6x 30.0
3 times a day, add 15 drops in a small glass of water and drink in small sips.

Also homeopathic remedies for the lymphatic system are important for the treatment of hemorrhoids. These remedies stimulate the excretion of acids, metabolic waste and toxins. They also purify and strengthen the function of the connective tissue from the blood vessels and stimulate the immune system.

Therefore you also should take one of the following remedies:

1) Badiaga 12x
For 4 weeks, 2 times a day, take 5 globules. Let them melt in your mouth.

2) Baryta carbonica 12x (Barium carbonicum D12)
For 4 weeks, 2 times a day, take 5 globules. Let them melt in your mouth.

3) Barium iodatum 12x (Barium jodatum D12)
For 4 weeks, 2 times a day, take 5 globules. Let them melt in your mouth.

4) Calcarea 12x (Calcium carbonicum D12)
For 4 weeks, 2 times a day, take 5 globules. Let them melt in your mouth.

5) Mercury solubilis 12x (Mercurius solubilis D12)
For 4 weeks, 2 times a day, take 5 globules. Let them melt in your mouth.

6) Thuja 12x
For 4 weeks, 2 times a day, take 5 globules. Let them melt in your mouth.

Hemorrhoids - Treatment and prevention with Schuessler salts

A defective metabolism favors hemorrhoids, a weak immune system and health problems, and is often the result of a disturbance of mineral distribution and mineral intake.

Although we may receive enough minerals in our food, in the event of a metabolic disorder, not all of the minerals may reach the cells. Deficiency of mineral salts weaken the immune system, disrupt the hormonal balance and slow down the metabolism.

Prerequisite to avoid hemorrhoids is a balanced acid-base-balance, proper nutrition and good blood circulation. Nutrition is a key factor in the treatment of our metabolism and health. With a balanced and varied diet the body will be supplied with all the necessary nutrients. The cells and organs are strengthened.

At the same time you support your immune system, your metabolism and ensure a perfect acid-base-balance, the foundation of our health and for the treatment of hemorrhoids. Proper nutrition also helps to extract toxins from the body and dissolves healing blockages.

Remember: There are several metabolic blockages which you have to treat for to deacidify and detoxify the body of people suffering from hemorrhoids.

Metabolic blockage No. 1: The acid-base balance

Too much sugar, white flour, meat and sausage acidifies the body. In order to neutralize the acids precious bases are consumed. What is not neutralized, ends up as a "hazardous waste" in the connective tissue and leads to its acidity.

The metabolic process slows down. We get hemorrhoids, gain weight despite calorie conscious diet and exercise.

Schuessler-salt No. 9 Sodium phosphate 6x (Nr. 9 Natrium phosphoricum D6) ensures that toxins and metabolic residues are flushed from the body. Sodium phosphate (Natrium phosphoricum) also stimulates the metabolism of fat and sugar degradation.

Metabolic blockage No. 2: The connective tissue

The connective tissue is more than just a connection between the organs. It serves as a nutrient storage and intermediate storage of metabolic products. In the connective tissue the cells dispose their waste products. That the toxins can leave the body, enough mineral salts must be present.

A mineral deficiency causes metabolic residues, acidification and overload with toxins. They remain in the connective tissue and bind water. It comes to hemorrhoids and water retention (edema) in the tissues of the body.

The salts No. 6 Potassium sulph 6x (Nr. 6 Kalium sulfuricum D6), No. 9 Sodium phosphate 6x (Nr. 9 Natrium phosphoricum D6), No. 10 Sodium sulphate 6x (Nr. 10 Natrium sulfuricum D6) and No. 11 Silicea 12x promote the excretion of acids and toxins through the skin and activate the detoxification via the liver, intestines and kidneys.

Metabolic blockage No. 3: The digestion

Environmental pollution, lush diet and medication burden the liver, our central metabolic organ. Stomach, pancreas and intestines suffer with. Many metabolic processes stalled and it comes to hemorrhoids, weight gain, constipation, bloating and stomach problems.

No. 4 Potassium chloratum 6x (Nr. 4 Kalium chloratum D6), No. 6 Potassium sulph 6x (Nr. 6 Kalium sulfuricum D6) and No. 10 Sodium sulphate 6x (Nr. 10 Natrium sulfuricum D6) give the liver and digestive organs new power. The metabolic processes accelerate. Toxins and acids are excreted faster.

Metabolic blockage No. 4: Our water Resources

Every day the organism produces acids and waste products that have to be filtered out by the kidneys. But part of it also ends up in the connective tissue, because for the removal mineral salts are absent. We get hemorrhoids.

No. 8 Sodium chloratum 6x (Nr. 8 Natrium chloratum D6) regulates the water balance and No. 10 Sodium sulphate 6x (Nr. 10 Natrium sulfuricum D6) drained. Together they controll the water balance in the body.

Metabolic blockage No. 5: The protein digestion

Protein is essential for the production of enzymes, hormones, muscles and the connective tissue. However, in the cleavage of proteins ammonia is formed (a strong cytotoxin). The liver converts the ammonia into non-toxic urea, which is excreted in the urine.

Therefore, a high intake of protein is a strong decontamination work for our two kidneys. Hemorrhoids are the result.

Salt No. 9 Sodium phosphate 6x (Nr. 9 Natrium phosphoricum D6) helps the body in protein metabolism. Salt No. 6 Potassium sulph 6x (Nr. 6 Kalium sulfuricum D6) supports the liver in the degradation of ammonia.

Metabolic blockage No. 6: The digestion of fat

We need fats because they provide essential fatty acids. But fat is also the best energy storage in times of need. The body hoards it especially in the thighs and hips, the abdomen and buttocks.

But the adipose tissue is also a deposit for toxins. This stimulates hemorrhoids.

The Schuessler salts No. 6 Potassium sulph 6x (Nr. 6 Kalium sulfuricum D6), No. 9 Sodium phosphate 6x (Nr. 9 Natrium phosphoricum D6) and No. 10 Sodium sulphate 6x (Nr. 10 Natrium sulfuricum D6) help to lead out the contaminants.

Metabolic blockage No. 7: The carbohydrate digestion

Carbohydrates are energy pure. But in abundance they are also responsible for weight gain and acidification of the body. What is not burned, will be converted and stored in fat. Especially sweets and white flour products are dangerous. They let the blood sugar level rise up rapidly. This leads to a strong insulin release.

Insulin normalizes blood sugar. At the same time burning fat is broken. Insulin leads fats from the meal in the fat stores of the body. In addition, it holds back water in the body and causes rapidly new hunger.

The Schuessler salt No. 4 Potassium chloratum 6x (Nr. 4 Kalium chloratum D6) supports the combustion of sugar. Important are also the salts No. 6 Potassium sulph 6x (Nr. 6 Kalium sulphuricum D6) and No. 10 Sodium sulphate 6x (Nr 10 Natrium sulfuricum D6).

The combination of these salts Nos. 4, 6, 8, 9, 10 and 11 has proven itself well in the treatment of acidification and overload with toxins. Dissolve from each cell salt 1 tablet in a small glass of hot water (all together in the same glass). Drink in small sips half an hour before or after eating.

After 6 weeks you make one week break, then repeat. If necessary, you can repeat this treatment several times.

Acute and inflamed hemorrhoids with pain:
No. 3 Ferrum phos 12x (Nr. 3 Ferrum phosphoricum D12) and
No. 4 Potassium chloratum 6x (Nr. 4 Kalium chloratum D6)
Alternate each remedy half-hourly by taking 2 tablets. Let them melt in your mouth.
In addition apply the biochemical ointment No. 4 Potassium chloratum (Nr. 4 Kalium chloratum)

To strengthen the connective tissue of the hemorrhoids:
Nr. 11 Silicea 12x and
No. 1 Calcium fluorite 12x (Nr. 1 Calcium fluoratum D12)
Alternate each remedy daily by taking 4 times a day 2 tablets. Let them melt in your mouth.

Hemorrhoids with itching:
No. 5 Potassium phosphate 6x (Nr. 5 Kalium phosphoricum D6)
No. 7 Magnesium phosphate 6x (Nr. 7 Magnesium phosphoricum D6) and
No. 11 Silicea 12x
Alternate each remedy daily by taking 4 times a day 2 tablets. Let them melt in your mouth.
In addition apply the biochemical ointments No. 5 Potassium phosphate, No. 7 Magnesium phosphate and No. 11 Silicea. Alternate the ointments daily.

Itching and cracks in the anus:
No. 3 Ferrum phos 12x (Nr. 3 Ferrum phosphoricum D12) and
No. 7 Magnesium phosphate 6x (Nr. 7 Magnesium phosphoricum D6)
Alternate each remedy hourly by taking 2 tablets. Let them melt in your mouth.

Stinging and nagging pain:
No. 7 Magnesium phosphate 6x (Nr. 7 Magnesium phosphoricum D6)
Half-hourly take 2 tablets. Let them melt in your mouth.

Chronic inflammation of the hemorrhoids:
No. 4 Potassium chloratum 6x (Nr. 4 Kalium chloratum D6) and
No. 6 Potassium sulph 6x (Nr. 6 Kalium sulfuricum D6)
Alternate each remedy daily by taking 4 times a day 2 tablets. Let them melt in your mouth.

Hemorrhoids with burning and stinging pain. Also, if constipation alternates with diarrhea:
No. 8 Sodium chloratum 6x (Nr. 8 Natrium chloratum D6)
No. 10 Sodium sulphate 6x (Nr. 10 Natrium sulfuricum D6) and
No. 3 Ferrum phos 6x (Nr. 3 Ferrum phosphoricum D6)
Alternate each remedy hourly by taking 2 tablets. Let them melt in your mouth.

Hemorrhoids with bleeding:
No. 11 Silicea 12x and
No. 2 Calcium phosphate 6x (Nr. 2 Calcium phosphoricum D6)
Alternate each remedy hourly by taking 2 tablets. Let them melt in your mouth.

Hemorrhoids with constipation and flatulence:
No. 7 Magnesium phosphate 6x (Nr. 7 Magnesium phosphoricum D6) and
No. 10 Sodium sulphate 6x (Nr. 10 Natrium sulfuricum D6)
Alternate each remedy hourly by taking 2 tablets. Let them melt in your mouth.

Hemorrhoids and constipation due to liver disease and a bitter taste in the mouth (often a weakness of pancreas and liver):
No. 10 Sodium sulphate 6x (Nr. 10 Natrium sulfuricum D6)
4 times a day, take 2 tablets, let them melt in your mouth.

Constipation and hemorrhoids:
No. 1 Calcium fluorite 12x (Nr. 1 Calcium fluoratum D12)
No. 9 Sodium phosphate 6x (Nr. 9 Natrium phosphoricum D6) and
No. 10 Sodium sulphate 6x (Nr. 10 Natrium sulfuricum D6)
Alternate each remedy daily by taking 4 times a day 2 tablets. Let them melt in your mouth.

Hemorrhoids and constipation due to colonic inertia:
No. 3 Ferrum phos 6x (Nr. 3 Ferrum phosphoricum D6)
No. 7 Magnesium phosphate 6x (Nr. 7 Magnesium phosphoricum D6)
No. 2 Calcium phosphate 6x (Nr. 2 Calcium phosphoricum D6) and
No. 9 Sodium phosphate 6x (Nr. 9 Natrium phosphoricum D6)
Alternate each remedy daily by taking 4 times a day 2 tablets. Let them melt in your mouth.

Biochemical health cure (Schuessler salts) for the treatment of chronic hemorrhoids and to strengthen the connective tissue of the hemorrhoids. Repeat 2 times.

1) No. 4 Potassium chloratum 6x (Nr. 4 Kalium chloratum D6)
The main means of all glands.
4 times a day, 2 tablets, let them melt in your mouth.
Alternating daily with the homeopathic remedy
Magnesium fluorite 6x (optimizes the effect of Potassium chloratum).
4 times a day, take 2 tablets, let them melt in your mouth.

2) After 3 weeks please take for 2 weeks:
No. 6 Potassium sulph 6x (Nr. 6 Kalium sulphuricum D6)
alternating daily with
No. 10 Sodium sulphate 6x (Nr. 10 Natrium sulphuricum D6)
4 times a day, take 2 tablets, let them melt in your mouth.

Another biochemical health cure (Schuessler salts) for the treatment of hemorrhoids and to strengthens the connective tissue of the hemorrhoids. Please take for 2 months:

Monday
No. 1 Calcium fluorite 12x (Nr. 1 Calcium fluoratum D12)
4 times a day, take 2 tablets, let them melt in your mouth.

Tuesday
No. 11 Silicea 12x
4 times a day, take 2 tablets, let them melt in your mouth.

Wednesday
No. 9 Sodium phosphate 6x (Nr. 9 Natrium phosphoricum D6)
4 times a day, take 2 tablets, let them melt in your mouth.

Thursday
No. 1 Calcium fluorite 12x (Nr. 1 Calcium fluoratum D12)
4 times a day, take 2 tablets, let them melt in your mouth.

Friday
No. 11 Silicea 12x
4 times a day, take 2 tablets, let them melt in your mouth.

Saturday
No. 1 Calcium fluorite 12x (Nr. 1 Calcium fluoratum D12)
4 times a day, take 2 tablets, let them melt in your mouth.

Sunday
No. 9 Sodium phosphate 6x (Nr. 9 Natrium phosphoricum D6)
4 times a day, take 2 tablets, let them melt in your mouth.

Biochemical health cure (Schuessler salts) for the treatment of painful and inflamed hemorrhoids. For 2 months, please take:

Monday
No. 3 Ferrum phos 12x (Nr. 3 Ferrum phosphoricum D12)
4 times a day, take 2 tablets, let them melt in your mouth.

Tuesday
No. 1 Calcium fluorite 12x (Nr. 1 Calcium fluoratum D12)
4 times a day, take 2 tablets, let them melt in your mouth.

Wednesday
No. 3 Ferrum phos 12x (Nr. 3 Ferrum phosphoricum D12)
4 times a day, take 2 tablets, let them melt in your mouth.

Thursday
No. 1 Calcium fluorite 12x (Nr. 1 Calcium fluoratum D12)
4 times a day, take 2 tablets, let them melt in your mouth.

Friday
No. 11 Silicea 12x
4 times a day, take 2 tablets, let them melt in your mouth.

Saturday
No. 3 Ferrum phos 12x (Nr. 3 Ferrum phosphoricum D12)
4 times a day, take 2 tablets, let them melt in your mouth.

Sunday
No. 1 Calcium fluorite 12x (Nr. 1 Calcium fluoratum D12)
4 times a day, take 2 tablets, let them melt in your mouth.
In addition apply the biochemical ointments No. 3 Ferrum phos and No. 1 Calcium fluorite. Alternate the ointments daily.

Biochemical health cure (Schuessler salts) for the treatment of hemorrhoids due to liver disease and sensitivity to changes in weather. Duration of intake: 2 months

Monday
No. 7 Magnesium phosphate 6x (Nr. 7 Magnesium phosphoricum D6)
4 times a day, take 2 tablets, let them melt in your mouth.

Tuesday
No. 10 Sodium sulphate 6x (Nr. 10 Natrium sulfuricum D6)
4 times a day, take 2 tablets, let them melt in your mouth.

Wednesday
No. 7 Magnesium phosphate 6x (Nr. 7 Magnesium phosphoricum D6)
4 times a day, take 2 tablets, let them melt in your mouth.

Thursday
No. 6 Potassium sulph 6x (Nr. 6 Kalium sulfuricum D6)
4 times a day, take 2 tablets, let them melt in your mouth.

Friday
No. 7 Magnesium phosphate 6x (Nr. 7 Magnesium phosphoricum D6)
4 times a day, take 2 tablets, let them melt in your mouth.

Saturday: No. 10 Sodium sulphate 6x (Nr. 10 Natrium sulfuricum D6)
4 times a day, take 2 tablets, let them melt in your mouth.

Sunday
No. 6 Potassium sulph 6x (Nr. 6 Kalium sulfuricum D6)
4 times a day, take 2 tablets, let them melt in your mouth.

Biochemical health cure (Schuessler salts) for the treatment of hemorrhoids due to indigestion, bloating, flatulence and dyspepsia. Duration of intake: 2 months

Monday
No. 7 Magnesium phosphate 6x
4 times a day, take 2 tablets, let them melt in your mouth.

Tuesday
No. 5 Potassium phosphate 6x (Nr. 5 Kalium phosphoricum D6)
4 times a day, take 2 tablets, let them melt in your mouth.

Wednesday
No. 7 Magnesium phosphate 6x
4 times a day, take 2 tablets, let them melt in your mouth.

Thursday
No. 9 Sodium phosphate 6x (Nr. 9 Natrium phosphoricum D6)
4 times a day, take 2 tablets, let them melt in your mouth.

Friday
No. 7 Magnesium phosphate 6x
4 times a day, take 2 tablets, let them melt in your mouth.

Saturday
No. 5 Potassium phosphate 6x (Nr. 5 Kalium phosphoricum D6)
4 times a day, take 2 tablets, let them melt in your mouth.

Sunday
No. 9 Sodium phosphate 6x (Nr. 9 Natrium phosphoricum D6)
4 times a day, take 2 tablets, let them melt in your mouth.

Biochemical health cure (Schuessler salts) to treat chronic hemorrhoids. Duration of intake: 3 months

Monday
No. 1 Calcium fluorite 12x (Nr. 1 Calcium fluoratum D12)
4 times a day, take 2 tablets, let them melt in your mouth.

Tuesday
No. 3 Ferrum phos 6x (Nr. 3 Ferrum phosphoricum D6)
4 times a day, take 2 tablets, let them melt in your mouth.

Wednesday
No. 5 Potassium phosphate 6x (Nr. 5 Kalium phosphoricum D6)
4 times a day, take 2 tablets, let them melt in your mouth.

Thursday
No. 1 Calcium fluorite 12x
4 times a day, take 2 tablets, let them melt in your mouth.

Friday
No. 7 Magnesium phosphate 6x (Nr. 7 Magnesium phosphoricum D6)
4 times a day, take 2 tablets, let them melt in your mouth.

Saturday
No. 1 Calcium fluorite 12x
4 times a day, take 2 tablets, let them melt in your mouth.

Sunday
No. 3 Ferrum phos 12x
4 times a day, take 2 tablets, let them melt in your mouth.

A biochemical health cure (Schuessler salts) to treat hemorrhoids, cardiovascular disorders and weakness of the heart. Duration: 2 months

Monday
No. 7 Magnesium phosphoricum 6x
4 times a day, take 2 tablets, let them melt in your mouth.

Tuesday
No. 5 Potassium phosphoricum 6x (Nr. 5 Kalium phosphoricum D6)
4 times a day, take 2 tablets, let them melt in your mouth.

Wednesday
No. 7 Magnesium phosphoricum 6x
4 times a day, take 2 tablets, let them melt in your mouth.

Thursday
No. 3 Ferrum phosphoricum 6x
4 times a day, take 2 tablets, let them melt in your mouth.

Friday
No. 7 Magnesium phosphoricum 6x
4 times a day, take 2 tablets, let them melt in your mouth.

Saturday
No. 5 Potassium phosphoricum 6x (Nr. 5 Kalium phosphoricum D6)
4 times a day, take 2 tablets, let them melt in your mouth.

Sunday
No. 3 Ferrum phosphoricum 6x
4 times a day, take 2 tablets, let them melt in your mouth.

More information about Schuessler salts you will find in my book:

Schuessler Salts - Homeopathic cell salts for your health

Epilogue

I hope that you have discovered a lot of new and interesting things while reading this book.

I wish you much success in the treatment of hemorrhoids with Homeopathy and Schuessler salts, joy in life and especially your health.

You will find more information about my books on my website.

Robert Kopf

Printed in Great Britain
by Amazon

21750539R00056